*Yvonne,
Keep smiling, keep striving and keep moving forward! Thank you for the and support.
Love,
Katie*

February 2010

Moving Forward

Katherine A. Butler

~ *Dedication* ~

Mom and Dad
Without your constant love; support; and encouragement that, I must admit, at times felt like nagging and got on my nerves, thank you. I would not be alive today without you.

Dr. Patti Dolan
It was the times when all hope seemed lost that you followed your intuition and we tried something new. Chemotherapy and all you helped to keep my spirits high and maintain this crazy sense of humor. Thank God for you on my team and for getting me off prednisone!

Dr. Manus Praserthdam
Thank you for never giving up on me and my kidneys! Prednisone may 'make young girl ugly' but that is what I needed to be here today. You are very wise and I am forever grateful.

Dr. Vitalis Unaeze
Two words that I will forever remember are 'Be Strong'. Through it all I could be no different. I will always keep that mischievous smile.

~ *Acknowledgments* ~

I would like to thank my family and friends for their unwavering love and support, without whom my survival would not have been possible. An extra special thank you to the following:

My brother, Joe, for always being there when I called and for always caring and making me laugh when I was in the worst mood.

Carol B. Robbins, for being a never-ending source of encouragement. For always believing in me and blessing my life daily, I thank you.

Myles E. Daniel for always believing in me as well as my dreams. From you I gain strength and wisdom to help me learn and grow. You make me smile, laugh and have given me wings to fly.

Vickie Harriman without whom I never would have finished this book and embarked on teaching others about *my story*.

Greg and Rachel Barteaux for the care packages and phone calls to keep my mind occupied and my spirits running high.

Kennedy Barteaux for sending me Mad Libs, listening to the absolute nonsense once they were completed and for always being there . . . even when things were at their worst.

Phyllis Bolduc for playing cards. For always being there to tell me things would get better, I would make it and to keep fighting...even when I was tired of doing so.

Marie Rorke for seeing me at every step of this journey and believing in miracles.

The staff of Gulfcoast Oncology at St. Anthony's Hospital in St. Petersburg, Florida: for keeping my spirits soaring and contributing to this crazy sense of humor. You kept me going.

A very special thank you and appreciation for the love and support shown from the individuals associated with **Conrad Mobile Home Park** in Seminole, Florida; **The Florida Winery** and **Merry Mouse** located at John's Pass in Madeira Beach, Florida; and **Bealls Department Store** located at the Largo Mall in Largo, Florida.

A great wedge in relationships is that we become over-occupied with making a living, gaining materialistic possessions, working hard, achieving our dreams, paying our bills and just getting things done that we lose sight on the finer things in life. These are 'tasks' and certainly not life's purpose. Our purpose is learning to love...ourselves, God and others. Take the time to share your love because one day it may be too late to do so.

~ A Note from the Author ~

First and foremost I need to thank you, the reader, for picking up this book. In the pages to follow you will learn about my personal journey with Systemic Lupus and how it has forever changed my life.

Lupus (Latin for wolf) is a complex auto-immune disease that, at times, takes years to diagnose. It affects everyone differently and within the same individual, your sense of what is 'normal' can change from day to day or week to week.

I can honestly say that what you will read is not sugar coated in any way and there will be some very raw emotions expressed at certain points. It will also describe ways for which I was able to maintain a sense of humor and gain strength and knowledge from each experience that occurred.

I hope that in some way this book will be an inspiration to at least one individual. A sense of peace and strength knowing that they are not going through this alone, there is a light at the end of the tunnel and that some days will absolutely be better than others.

Please remember that things could always be worse and we are certainly tested in this life but never given more than what we are able to handle. Move forward with an open mind and heart.

Katherine A. Butler

~ *The Wolf* ~

It was there for years.
Pacing,
lurking,
watching,
cowardly afraid
to attack outright.

Staying close to home
we sought help.
None came.

Every event
was isolated.
Shielded
from the history.
Unacknowledged.
Dismissed.

More shallow attacks,
more symptoms,
more evidence,
more unanswered questions,
more opportunities
come and go.

Traveling hours away
we sought help.
None came.

It's all in your head.
Depression.
Panic.
Lazy.
Hypochondriac.
Have some medications.

Then it struck!
Moving swiftly,
quietly,
no more pacing
or lurking.
An attack for the kill.

Striking each system,
going for the organs,
shredding
everything
in its path.

Piece by piece
breaking it down
the time had come:
diagnosis or death.

The wolf attacked,
shown his face,
one final time.

7 MOVING FORWARD

Finally a relief
comes with fear,
confusion,
anger,
more questions
and a sense of hope.

Diagnosis: Lupus

The strong
and determined
shall survive.

The wolf will not conquer,
for I will prevail.

~ *The Life I Was Living* ~

It was the best year of my life! I was living my dreams, having a blast and cruising along as if nothing could go wrong and everything was right with the world. Not that I was naive because I had definitely seen some turbulent times in my twenty-eight years but, for the moment, everything seemed to be fitting into place. Even if it was only for a moment...that moment was priceless.

The year was 2006 and the adventures were endless. I started the year working as a manager of a chocolate shop in the small town of Skowhegan, Maine and had just wrapped up the busy holiday season. I had the opportunity to take part in everything from actually making and packaging some of the candy to greeting the customers and making sure all shipments were to arrive safely and on time. Being the manager, I also had the responsibilities of taking care of the cash register, making sure deposits were made each day and that we had enough change available without having to go to the bank in the middle of the day.

I had grown up in the town right next to Skowhegan, called Norridgewock, which was even smaller and, for the most part, everyone knew a major part of someone else's business. I had come back to the area after being away at college and different homes I had been renting for almost eight years. At this point in my life, I was doing no work related to either of my college degrees: an associate degree in nursing and a bachelor of science degree in biology but, I was having a good time and learning more in other areas of interest such as writing, history and travel.

I celebrated Maine Maple Sunday at the sugar camp with family and friends for a wonderful pig roast and gathering in Searsmont, Maine. I was enrolled in as well as completed a fifteen-week poetry writing class through Skowhegan Area High School's Adult Education program. This course challenged its students to think beyond the normal realm of their writing, explore different topics to write about as well as learn from a variety of poets and their styles. We also learned that each draft of our writing had something valuable to contribute to the finished product and overall growth and development as a writer. At the end we had a presentation open to the public and it was the first time I had done any form of public speaking since I was in high school and a part of the speech team. I also became more interested and involved in politics, actually attending a rally as well as spending primary election night in Lewiston, Maine at one of the campaign parties in the race for governor.

By the last weekend in March, I had taken off to our nation's capital for a long weekend with friends for Cherry Blossom Festival. It was the first time I had really gone on a trip without my family and I was excited about the adventure. We toured monuments, walked around the trees in full bloom, stayed up to all hours of the night. I relearned history and even went to the circus. I spent time everywhere from China Town to Little Italy in Baltimore to Arlington National Cemetery watching the changing of the guards at the Tomb of the Unknown. Never once, even in the city, did I feel unsafe. Arlington definitely had the most profound impact on me during that trip. There was a funeral going on at the time that we were there and we were unable to get over to where President Kennedy was buried. However, I do remember standing atop one of the hills and just looking across at all of the white stones lined up. It was the realization of what my freedom has cost and how I ungratefully had been taking it for granted. I took in everything I could during my time in Washington and vowed that I would return some day to continue that quest.

The end of April I was off again, this time to Las Vegas. Eight of us from different parts of the country came together for a few days of endless fun and excitement. They had adopted me, not legally, into their hearts and family and we were coming together for a long weekend. My role on this trip was to not only have a wonderful time but also to take care of a four and a half year old boy, the son of a couple who were on the trip. It had been twenty years since I had last seen the Vegas strip and this time my folks were not with me. We stayed at the Venetian, took in the canal shops and Circus Circus, walked to Caesar's Palace, the Wynn and frequented Haagen-Dazs Ice Cream Shop and the pool. There was nothing like waking up to a four and a half year old opening the curtains, still on Milwaukee time, and saying loud enough for us all to hear: "it's almost morning!" The best souvenirs that I came home with being the precious memories to last a lifetime.

While still racing on the adrenaline from my trips, I purchased a 2006 Mazda Tribute and decided it was time to move on from the small town seclusion. The last week in May I gave my notice at the chocolate shop and started focusing on a *summer job* that I had known and loved. I was returning to work in a health center at a co-ed camp for seven to fifteen year olds along the shores of Crescent Lake in Casco, Maine. It would be my fifth year there and this place was my second home and the staff was like family. Campers I had seen coming for years and watching them grow, blessed with the opportunity to be a part of their lives, even if only for four weeks a summer.

When camp ended, I moved back home and announced to my family that in one week I would be leaving for Florida. At first, they believed this was another one of my random trips to continue the adventures of my year thus far. I then told them that when I left, I would be traveling down Labor Day weekend and I was *moving* to Florida...no job, the opportunity to stay at a friend's house in Winter Springs until I could find something and with what little money I had saved throughout the summer. I was picking up and moving forward or, in this case, moving south.

When I left, I was leaving behind all that I had known and grown up with. My family and I had traveled quite a bit while growing up; however, I knew no other home than in the state of Maine. I wanted a fresh start. I wanted to go to a place where I didn't know but just a few people, make new friends as well as

MOVING FORWARD

learn and grow as an individual. Moving away, I did not fit into a certain role among family and friends and I could become my own person. It was time to spread my wings and leave the nest. I was in a position where I felt comfortable knowing that if I were to fall I could get back up again and, if by the grace of God, I spread my wings and soared, even better.

I arrived in Florida and settled in while looking for work. I found a sales job in Orlando which, I must admit; I knew nothing about and decided it was better than nothing and certainly a learning opportunity. Throughout my time there I worked six days a week and sometimes more than fifteen hours per day. I went on four different road trips: Vero Beach; Daytona Beach twice; and to Augusta, Georgia. The second road trip to Daytona Beach was a Toys for Tots drive and I was actually in charge of making sure things ran smoothly. Okay, so it was a rough trip from the start and the only thing that actually ran smoothly were the people I met while I was there. One man, in particular, was willing to help me out with my sales skills or lack thereof. He worked in the building where I had set up my location and we saw each other throughout the week. He talked about pitch lines, when to stop talking and close the deal as well as conversations about general life and what had brought me to the area. He has become a wonderful friend in the time since.

The middle of November my world was starting to crumble. I wasn't feeling right and it *wasn't* homesickness. Something was seriously wrong but I couldn't figure out what. I had been to a local emergency room a couple of times and told I had everything from bronchitis and pneumonia to whooping cough and pancreatitis. It got to the point I had to stop working, pack my things and move to the Gulf Coast to where my parents had retired since my moving down Labor Day weekend. I felt that the greatest thing I would be losing would be my independence during, what I liked to call, a brief transitional period.

I ended up in the emergency room more than once and was still given different diagnoses, a variety of medications and no clear cut reason other than I was just overworked and not sleeping enough. If only a little extra sleep could have solved all the complications that were yet to arise and prevent the world from caving in around me.

13 MOVING FORWARD

~ The Missing Piece ~

It was the morning of February 6, 2007. I had already been at work for three hours at the local gym and was scheduled to return in less than six. I was working a split-shift to cover hours for a coworker on vacation. I felt okay when I arrived at four that morning and the only noticeable difference between that and any other morning was that my legs were swollen and I had some difficulty climbing the stairs. For days now my legs had been swollen and I had attributed it to being tired and on my feet all day. When I left the house that morning, still living with my parents during that brief transitional period, Dad had already warned me that if the swelling had not gone down by the time I returned home on my break they were going to take me to the emergency room. The past couple nights the swelling had not been decreasing when I elevated my legs for hours and I knew it wasn't promising that they were going to decrease in size while running around on cement floors at the gym. When I arrived home a little after seven in the morning my folks stood true to their words and drove me, as I was complaining the entire time, to a local emergency room yet again. Little did we know something major was wrong and we knew even less of what to expect.

The nurse had drawn blood and did urine tests, even though I told them straight out I wasn't taking drugs, did not drink and was definitely *not* pregnant. Just standard testing was what I was told. An EKG was performed to check my heart, I was on constant blood pressure monitoring and an ultrasound of my legs was completed to look for blood clots. Everything I had done was ordered with immediate results and we found out I was going to be admitted within a half hour of arriving. Seriously, I did not have time for that in my schedule. I had to return to work for my afternoon shift and furthermore, I had no health insurance coverage at the time.

Within the hour, we learned I was being diagnosed with acute renal failure, congestive heart failure, hypertension and a bacterial infection. They knew what I had but there was no idea of the cause.

As I laid in the emergency room, I could feel the life drain out of me. I was exhausted. The more doctors and nurses tried to talk with me the more tired I became. I don't know if it was the pain medication they gave me or just my condition at the time but I went to sleep. When I woke up, consciously anyway, it was late afternoon and I was in the Intensive Care Unit (ICU). I had a blood pressure of about 230 over 140. I had lost ten pounds since October 2006 but within four days prior to this moment I had gained eight pounds back. Mom and Dad were told that there were many possible causes. One of them was positive HIV. It could be a variety of auto-immune diseases or it could be an endless list of words that just made them worry more. Time will tell, just be patient is what they were told and more testing would be done.

My first night in ICU I missed dinner but it was not too late to order something and have it delivered specially to the room. For some reason, a grilled cheese sandwich sounded good. Sounding good was about as far as it went because when it arrived that was the worst looking sandwich I had ever seen. How can you mess up a grilled cheese sandwich? I didn't even know that was possible! I don't know if someone in the kitchen was mad they had to make it or this is the way they all looked coming out of the kitchen. No matter which, I couldn't eat it. Maybe I was just tired and cranky from being at the hospital all day. The grease dripping out of it was enough to kill anyone and the look of it alone was enough to make me nauseous. Instead I sent my father out for cinnamon sticks. At least they were edible. Never in the time since have I ordered a grilled cheese sandwich while I was in the hospital.

Numerous doctors and staff were coming in and out of my room. To start with, I attempted to listen to every detail they were saying. They came in with information about what could possibly

15   MOVING FORWARD

be wrong, asking more questions about different symptoms I may have noticed and attempting to outline a treatment plan. The only symptoms that I had noticed leading up to this admission were my legs swelling and I was a little more tired than usual. Neither one of those truly alarmed me and I went about my days doing normal activities. I have no idea how many times I repeated that same information to a variety of people. It soon boiled down to knowing I had a serious condition, becoming confused and then just plain tuning them all out. I really didn't have the energy to care about all they were saying. I just knew I did not have time to be there and needed to find some way of getting back home and back to work.

After being stabilized, I had a kidney biopsy on the 8th of February. From there it was determined I only had 28 percent function. I should mention that back on January 16 and 17, less than a month prior; I went to a different local hospital three times with similar symptoms and sent home each time with a different diagnosis and combination of medications. I was diagnosed with hematuria, an enlarged spleen, enlarged lymph nodes, anemia and an allergic reaction to medications they had previously prescribed all within a matter of my three visits. I was also told that there was decreased kidney function at that time. Its cause was unknown; however, due to not having any health insurance I would not be admitted. Believe me, if you know something is wrong, get a second opinion! Seek a second opinion because it is your life, not theirs!

Everyday I was having numerous blood tests, CT scans and x-rays of everything from my chest and abdomen to ultrasounds and echocardiograms. There had to be something, other than sleep, to pass the time in the intensive care unit and being wheeled around to different tests seemed to be the answer. I think the only part of me they didn't officially test were my eye lashes because everywhere else felt poked and prodded about a million times.

February 12 it came back that I had a positive ANA test and the following day I had a confirmed diagnosis of Systemic Lupus Erythematosus (SLE). Finally a diagnosis! It wasn't that I knew exactly what I was dealing with but it was a start. It was something I could live with and work with. For years I had been told all of these symptoms were in my head, I was making them up. It was after I had a diagnosis and reviewed the criteria I was able to trace symptoms back. It was a disease that had been lurking in my system for as far back as twelve years.

Lupus, for me, was like a jigsaw puzzle. I received one piece of information at a time, one symptom, one single reason for a trip to the doctor. Then there came that moment when I finally was holding the magic piece. It was the one that closed the gaps and united all the pieces of the previous years. There was no more treating me for low blood sugar levels; depression; telling me it was *all in my head*; or even random pancreatitis that the previous doctors had contributed to my drinking, even though I didn't drink. There was no more just treating a symptom but the cause of all that had been and those that were to come. It was the one piece that not only brought me to the greatest challenge of my life but it gave me the determination to conquer that challenge. I finally had a diagnosis I could live with.

17 MOVING FORWARD

~ *A Look Back* ~

Once I had a confirmed diagnosis of lupus, my parents and I were able to go back and begin filling in the pieces. This diagnosis was the answer to all of the clues that had been lurking within my system for years. As far back as I can remember I have had a high level of sensitivity to sun exposure. It did not appear to matter what level of SPF protection I used or how many times throughout the day I applied it...I would always burn, blister and peel. It was also quite common for my skin to appear blotchy over the entire exposed area.

For many years my hands and feet would swell and I attributed it to the heat and humidity. When they would get cold, my fingers and toes as well as hands and feet would turn bright white, then blue, and as they would begin to warm again they would turn bright red and be throbbing. I believed everyone's hands and feet did this. I did not realize that it could actually be a symptom of Raynaud's Syndrome, a vascular disorder that affects blood flow to the extremities.

I also had extreme episodes of thinning hair, to the point that I actually had patches where there was literally no hair on my head. Luckily, I had thick hair to start with so it was not quite as noticeable to others. To me; however, it was very disturbing. It would come out in clumps, even with just running my fingers through it. Showers made it worse so I took a lot of baths for a while and brushing it would just leave clumps in the bristles. These phases would come and go, usually lasting eight to twelve weeks at a time.

It was during the summer of 1995, while attending a medical forum at Simmons College in Boston; I was taken to Beth Israel Hospital and diagnosed with ruptured ovarian cysts. I had an eventful year in 1996 as well. I was finally off to college, for the first time, and was quickly diagnosed with migraines. I was further diagnosed with hypoglycemia after episodes of *passing out* and periods of great confusion. I had to continually test my blood sugar levels and most of the time they were within normal range. Everything was controlled with diet and exercise which did not always work out well at college. There was something about college life that the level of exercise decreased and the consumption of junk food increased. Occasionally I had a level in the low 50's and then had to adjust what I was eating and drink some juice.

I also began noticing that my hip and knee joints would make a popping sound while I walked. They would be sore and inflamed. It would not happen all the time; however, enough of it that my mother did not like walking beside me because of the sound.

In 2001, when I began working at summer camp, I noticed that for a few weeks I would run a fever as high as 102.0 degrees Farenheit. There was no explanation for the fevers and the only other symptoms I could have attributed with it were tiredness and headaches. Honestly, I took these symptoms with the wonderful experience of camp life itself. With my active schedule and the joy of watching campers at their activities, when I was not working in the health center, I attributed it to dehydration and limited amounts of sleep. No matter what the cause, I loved camp and it was not enough to keep me down.

The first time I was diagnosed with acute pancreatitis was back in August 2003 and I was told that I needed to stop drinking alcohol. That was not the cause, I did not drink, but doctors refused to search further for any other underlying causes. Pancreatitis, for me, has occurred six or seven times since this original diagnosis and I am treated with a BRAT (bananas, rice, applesauce and toast) diet and a great deal of rest.

A month later, in September 2003, I began to have seizure-like activity. There was no warning of when the episode would occur so they took place in many different, inconvenient locations: while walking up or down stairs; in the bathtub; while cooking dinner and places like that. Because of this, I was unable to drive anywhere for many months and had very limited use of such appliances as the stove.

While still on Tegretol, a medication to suppress seizure activity, the seizures began occurring with greater frequency and duration. In addition to that, one of the side effects was hallucinations. I was sent to Brigham and Women's hospital in Boston for further testing. After a few days of monitoring it was determined that the seizures were not affecting the brain activity and I had a new diagnosis of pseudo-seizures. There was one lesion discovered on the frontal lobe of my brain at this time through a MRI. It had an unknown cause and I was sent back to Maine, without treatment, due again to not having any health insurance.

The beginning of February 2004 I was diagnosed with depression and conversion disorder. At the time, I was living in northern Maine and had recently moved to Fort Kent from Madawaska. I had gone from working on an adult psychiatric unit to a nursing home to working in a call center for MBNA to eventually not being able to work at all due to my medical condition. I mention this because when I was diagnosed with depression and conversion disorder I was admitted to the same adult psychiatric unit that I had previously worked on. This time I was on the wrong side of the door and without the key! My first couple days of admission I was not allowed to have such things as even a pen or notebook in my room for fear by the staff, which were former coworkers, of injuring myself.

My last pseudo-seizure occurred on March 10, 2004. Interestingly enough, this was also the day that I left Fort Kent, Maine, walking out and literally moving out of the house, stress and confinements of an abusive relationship. I did not understand the tremendous amount of stress and another person's control I was under until it was no longer weighing me down. I have not had to take any medication since June 2004 for seizures, depression or conversion disorder.

As wonderful and exciting as 2006 was for travel and adventure, it also became a challenging year medically. Before moving to Florida I was diagnosed with an underactive thyroid and started on medication. I also received a letter from Coral Blood Services lab in California. The last time I donated a pint of blood for the American Red Cross they were unable to use it for a patient in need. I was told there was a clinically significant presence of an unknown antibody in my blood. I followed up with my primary care physician and was reassured that, even with the presence of this antibody, there was no effect on my overall health.

Throughout the summer and fall I noticed a marked increase in the amount of fluid intake I would have within a twenty-four hour period of time. I would constantly carry around my two liter camelback or thirty-two ounce Nalgene bottle filled with water. It was common for me to drink three plus liters of fluid per day.

About two months after moving to Florida, November 2006, I was diagnosed with a respiratory infection, bronchitis, possible whooping cough and another episode of pancreatitis. Three months later, I had the missing piece and my journey began.

21 MOVING FORWARD

~ *The Journey Begins* ~

Upon being diagnosed with Lupus, the challenge then became learning all I could about the disease. Questions flooded my mind. My parents turned from asking me to asking my brother, Joe, their questions. He was seventeen hundred miles away, in Southern Maine, would look up information and call back. I honestly do not know how many calls and hours of conversation they had. The more they spoke the more questions and concerns arose. What was the cause? What was the prognosis? What were the treatments? Would I be dependent? Could I return to work? Would I even make it out of the intensive care unit?

Shortly after diagnosis I understood the seriousness of it all when Joe took off work and showed up for a week vacation. As grateful as I was for his visit, I was more frustrated by the fact I spent his entire week down here in the hospital. He did keep me laughing and I would ask the most random questions about life beyond the white walls. Questions that included what did real food taste like, could he keep the crazy roommates away and, of course, if he could bust me out of there and we could go to the beach. As usual, the week went by too fast and by the time I got discharged he was already 1700 miles away again.

It was suggested that I apply for Medicaid and Social Security Disability Insurance. In a matter of days I had gone from running around not even taking a vitamin to lying in a hospital bed taking thirty-two pills per day. Without a doubt, I was told, I would be out of work for at least a year.

I would be doing a disservice to people if I did not first mention: find yourself an advocate. Someone who will be there to stand up for you, fight your battles, make phone calls, take notes at doctor's appointments, and make sure everything that needs to be done gets done. I am not saying that laziness comes with this but, honestly, I did not have the strength or endurance to do it all myself and the mental capacity and comprehension to remember it all was not there either. My mother became my advocate.

One of my most awakening moments was the day that I had to walk, okay hobble, into the social security office. I knew why I was there and that I needed the assistance but that was one of the hardest things that I had done to date. I felt degraded. Never did I believe at twenty-eight years old I would be looking for assistance from the government...just to survive. I felt so incompetent with my own abilities. I looked at the people around me and wondered how on earth I had gone from where I was a few months ago to sitting in that office waiting to speak with a representative.

With me I carried two three-inch binders full of medical information and that was just from the time I had been diagnosed, less than two months prior. Every test, report, notes and anything I could get my hands on about my case was in those binders. I didn't know how the system worked and it was like I thought they were going to read through it all and make a decision that day or something. Wrong. They didn't even want that information. Anything that was submitted had to come directly from my doctors. My personal information was taken and I was sent home to wait. Wait for a response to see if I could get any form of health insurance, if there was any assistance available that I qualified for and if I would survive the expenses that were already vastly accumulating. I just had to wait.

Surprisingly to me, I was approved for disability with my first application. I knew I was bad off and although I was relieved for the assistance, I was struck with the realization that I was *that* bad off. What did they not expect me to live or something? The worst hadn't even taken place yet as I would quickly come to learn! I had heard the stories of people having to wait and wait, making appeals for their cases and praying that someone would give them a break. Some assistance to help them just get the basic necessities for living. I thank God every day that my assistance came through when it did.

23 MOVING FORWARD

At the time of diagnosis, I was on five different medications for blood pressure. One of them was metoprolol. Honestly, it was a medication that messed with my head! The dreams that I would have very quickly turned into nightmares. Everything was either so horrific that I woke up screaming, literally, or so bizarre that there was no way it could be comprehended to occur in real life. Every time I fell asleep these dreams would take place, if only a twenty minute nap. It got to the point that, for a while, I was afraid to even close my eyes.

I would dream of the house being on fire while I was trapped in it because of my limited ability to move. I would be screaming for help, I have been told I was screaming out loud at times, with nobody coming to rescue me. Unfortunately, I would wake up with the reflection of the sun shining into my room which screwed me up even more. I thought that I had woken up but the sunlight turned into flames for the first few seconds.

I would dream of drowning. Not just like diving into some water or a boat capsizing and drowning that way. I would dream of having weights tied to me so I literally could not come to the surface. I would awaken, startled and gasping for breath, like it had actually occurred.

One time I dreamed of being up in Alaska with one of my friends when we started getting chased by polar bears. Not a very welcoming thought! As it played out we ended up at the beach, which was an even crazier thought because the polar bears were still chasing us in addition to Bengal tigers. I had never before thought of these two species coexisting, let alone coexisting to chase my friend and me across everything from the tundra to the tropics.

It was a process of learning as I went. Some days were definitely better than others and more productive as well. I learned to adjust my schedule to my abilities and work from there. I learned to keep things on a strict schedule and to alter my diet away from the foods I was *restricted* from having, such as cheese and tomato sauce, which I love. You will learn later in the story that it didn't always work out and, as my health improved, I came to learn that all foods were okay in moderation. I must admit that I was also easier to get along with once I learned that I could have foods I actually enjoyed.

25 MOVING FORWARD

~ *The Team* ~

When first admitted to the hospital I had more doctors than I could keep track of. People would come in and go out at all hours, some looking familiar and some not. Before long I was weaned down to only the ones necessary for my case. This core of doctors became my 'team' and the ones that I embraced and entrusted with my life...literally.

My primary care doctors became Jae Shin and Vitalis Unaeze. They were both hospitalists and a part of the same medical group. Within four months it was Dr. Unaeze and his physician assistant, Joanne. Through everything, the two words that Dr. Unaeze would tell me were 'Be Strong'. He even wrote it out on a piece of paper for me to look at during the roughest trials of my journey. I had to be strong, the alternative wasn't *consistently* appealing. Believe me, there were moments and even days that any alternative seemed more appealing. Fortunately, they were not overwhelmingly consistent and I could see some possible hope through the trial.

As for my nephrologist, I have been blessed with Dr. Manus Praserthdam. He is the primary reason why I am still alive today. When he first saw me, I had renal failure and was dumping more than five grams of protein in my urine within a twenty-four-hour period of time. To give some perspective, I was to be dumping no more than 100 *milligrams* per day. He was a source of strength and inspiration for not only me but to my parents as well. Encouraging me every step of the way, he would tell me not to worry and he would fix me. When I was on high doses of prednisone and looking like a chipmunk, it was Dr. Praserthdam that would tell me 'Prednisone make young girl ugly' and that always made me laugh. How honest that statement was! It was what I needed to survive and save the function of my kidneys so I had to find some humor to the nasty side effects. I trusted whatever decision he made regarding my course of treatment and still do. He has seen me through every step of the way and has always had my best interest in mind.

Dr. Patti Dolan became my hematologist and is a vital asset to maintaining my sense of humor, as crazy as it may be, and strength. She has treated me for everything from low red and white blood cell counts to guiding me through treatments of a blood clot during the time of other complications. She has overseen weekly blood work, 'happy meals' of fluid when I become dehydrated and chemotherapy infusions that I referred to as the only cocktail they would allow me to have. She is also the primary reason for me being able to wean down off prednisone as quickly as I did. It was causing muscle neuropathy (weakness) and got to the point that I ended up in a wheelchair. Little did we know, at the time, it was also deteriorating my bones.

The rheumatologist that I was provided with at the time of my diagnosis, I have not seen since March 2008. Not because it wasn't necessary to have an appointment, but I had been *dismissed* during the time of my brain infection in May 2007. When I had my first hip replacement, I was told that due to the fact I was seeing a rheumatologist in Gainesville, she would only ask for an update about once per year. I have kept in some contact with her because when I am admitted to the local hospital, she is the one that will be called upon. As for seeing her, I don't.

My team of doctors is what has kept me alive. I entrusted them with my life, the very air I was breathing, and am forever thankful that they have come with many blessings, much healing and lessons for my learning. They made it possible to keep smiling and keep fighting.

27 MOVING FORWARD

~ Learning As We Go ~

The interesting part about lupus is that it affects everyone differently and what may work for an individual one day does not necessarily mean that it will the following day. It was a game of trial and error, an obstacle course that occasionally had a landmine to take us completely off course and the doctors had to work even harder to get me back on track.

When first diagnosed I kept track of everything I ate, what challenges I faced throughout each day and what hours I would take naps. I had a very poor appetite and unless it was considered *finger foods*: such as grapes, toast or dry cereal, I was by no means interested in looking at it. In addition to that, I had been placed on a renal diet with sodium, potassium and protein restriction as well as it having to be low fat and low cholesterol. For challenges that I kept track of, it could have been anything from nausea and difficulty with my balance to joint pain, hand and foot cramping or simply breaking down emotionally. I liked to call those break downs my *moments* because I never knew what would trigger one or how long it would last. I was completely frustrated and overwhelmed at the beginning.

There was a great deal of time in the beginning that I felt like I was waffling: the inside of my body felt like it was literally shaking, I was off balance and could not concentrate or comprehend my surroundings. My blood pressure was taken three times a day sitting, standing and lying down. I did not only have a restriction on the foods I could eat, I also had a limit on the amount of fluid I could consume in a day as not to over work my kidneys. Because of the kidney damage at the time I was diagnosed, I also had to keep track of how many times I went to the bathroom to make sure my system was functioning properly.

My entire world changed. I now had a calendar with daily blocks larger than my cell phone so I could get all of the information to fit. Everything I did in the run of a day was recorded so I could go back and reflect on it later. This was helpful as my memory had turned to mush and if someone asked me what I did I was lucky to remember five minutes prior to the conversation. When I left the house I would joke that I had to carry a diaper bag full of stuff without having a child. I had to make sure I had a mask because of my weakened immune system; I needed snacks and drinks, a blanket and pillow in case I got exhausted and a sweatshirt because I could not maintain a normal body temperature and was always cold. I always carried a change of clothes with me for those *just in case* moments. Two things that I could not forget, especially living in Florida, were to carry sun block and a hat. I needed to carry around my thermometer, blood pressure cuff and a notebook. Most of the times I left the house I also had my list of medications, dosages and times that I took them as well as the latest blood work results in case our adventure ended with a trip to the emergency room or the doctor's office.

  I thought that when I was diagnosed was going to be the rough patch and now that I knew what I had it would be smooth sailing from there. I believed that complications would be few to none and I could go back living my life the way I had known, the way I had loved. Little did we know what was in store just a few months after that fateful trip to the emergency room in February.

~ *The Storm* ~

For a while now the headaches had been intensifying in severity as well as frequency. Things began to be blurry at times and I could barely hold my attention long enough to eat a cookie. Words were becoming confusing for me as well. I knew what I wanted to say; however, there was a miscommunication between my brain and my mouth that made things come out jumbled or completely off topic. Being diagnosed with Lupus for only three months I had no idea what was happening within me but I knew it wasn't right. Something needed to be done and soon because the more time that went by the worse I felt.

I was admitted to the hospital on May 24, 2007. I was not digesting anything and had to be started on intravenous fluids and antibiotics at that time. Having poor veins to begin with, I chose to go with a central line placement. A central line, or central venous catheter, is a catheter placed, for me, into the jugular vein of the neck with three access lines. They could give me all the fluids they needed to, including a couple units of blood, and draw my daily labs without repeatedly having to stick me like a voodoo doll. Seriously, I felt like a voodoo doll sometimes.

On May 31st, I had a MRI that showed a small lesion on the frontal lobe of my brain, a brain infection with an unknown cause. I was started on intravenous antibiotics of Rocephin. The treatment would last longer than my admission and I needed to be certain to have vascular access through a vein large enough to handle the heavy doses. On June 8th my central line was removed and a mediport was placed, which I still have to this day. A mediport (or port-a-cath) is different than a central line because it is surgically implanted beneath the skin of my chest with no exterior access. There is a small septum covered with silicone rubber that, when pierced, through the skin and into this septum, by a needle will access the reservoir. When the needle is removed, the reservoir covering reseals itself.

While waiting for surgery, to have the mediport placed, I had the craziest out-of-body experience. I saw myself lying on the stretcher. Things were happening in my mind just moments before it would happen in reality. At one point I just looked at my nurse, totally confused and said "I've done this already." Luckily they did not admit me to a different floor for further evaluation. I did not know if it was the infection, the medications or a combination. At the time I could not explain it or tell anyone about it because then I really would be considered nutty!

A couple of doctors that arrived on my team during this time were from infectious disease. They oversaw the antibiotic infusions for the infection. It was never determined if the infection was viral, fungal or what caused it. The greatest challenge that I had with them was due to their times of visit while I was in the hospital: anywhere between midnight and two in the morning. Regardless of the infection, which was in my brain, their visits barely woke me enough to comprehend who was there and answer the questions that they asked. It certainly did not stir me enough to relay the information to my parents the following morning when they came to visit.

One night, my father waited and waited for one of them to come in. When they did arrive, after midnight, my father was not in the most receptive of moods. Although they were busy, there was no reason for them to come in and wake me up. To expect me to remember information and be able to translate it in the morning was beyond my level of capabilities at the time. Dad told them that they were avoiding the family members and avoiding answering any questions that arose because of their *inconsiderate* time of coming in. This was not the only *discussion* that my father had with the doctors from infectious disease; however, it obviously made a lasting impression because the remainder of their visits were before ten-thirty in the evening!

June 2007 was my worst month for hospital stay time. I was inpatient a total of twenty-four days. I asked for frequent flyer miles and if I could have my own suite developed because of the long periods of time I seemed to be hanging around. The hospital became the only place I was allowed to go for vacation for any length of time.

Due to my weakness from the brain infection in combination with muscle neuropathy as a result of consistently high doses of Prednisone and intravenous Solu-Medrol I was at great risk for falls. I was placed on bed rest and in turn developed a blood clot in my left leg. Doctors would not treat it with blood thinners because of my brain infection and the risk of 'bleeding out'. Physical Therapy refused to work with me to gain strength due to the blood clot. It was a vicious cycle and I could only imagine running the circles within my mind. My body went from aching because of the infection and medications to aching because it longed to move. An IVC filter was placed to prevent the clot from moving into my lungs.

By the time of my next MRI, I had gone from having the one lesion on my frontal lobe to having that one in addition to ten lesions on the cerebellum. I kept the Rocephin and added Vancomycin. We then learned it was the Rocephin that was causing high fevers and switched it to Promaxim.

It got to the point that I could literally and honestly say that I did not care. There were nights when I would be laying in the hospital bed with tears running down my face and praying to God to die. I was done. I couldn't take it anymore. This wasn't living. I wanted to go back home, to Maine, to see my family and friends. To see my brother again was my ultimate goal. I wanted to die in peace. I also knew full well that if I was to travel to Maine, it might be the trip itself that killed me.

When I went downstairs for one of my MRIs maintenance was just beginning to work on one of the elevators. Unfortunately, it was the only elevator in that section to get from the main hospital over to the MRI room. By the time my test was completed the elevator was out of service. The challenge presented was to either be wheeled around outside to get around the building and go in a different entrance or attempt to climb the eleven stairs between me and level where I needed to be to easily make my way back to my room. Completely against the idea of being wheeled around outside in the condition I looked, I opted for the challenge. I decided the stairs would be great with the help of the railing, a guy from transport and my father. I was wrong. Halfway up, I was asked if I thought I could make it all the way. Are you kidding me?! There was no way I was going to attempt to turn around and go back down what progress I had already made. Tears and all I made it to the top of the stairs. I did not want anyone to talk with me, to make noise around me or to even look at me. I wanted to be completely left *alone*.

Unknown to me at the time, astronauts were working on the space station. From my hospital room I could look out at night and see two orange colored lights. It honestly looked like the two lights were in combat with each other. Maybe that is because I grew up watching the original *Star Wars* trilogy.

Night after night I would stay awake, starring out the window. I did not know what they were but they most certainly caught my attention and intrigued me. I consistently told Mom and Dad each day that I had seen them again and about the so-called combats. I got the "uh-huh" and confused looks. One morning, about one-thirty, I called home. I have come to learn that this is never a good time to call, especially if you are calling from the hospital, regardless of the brain infection. I made my father literally get up and go outside. I never figured out if he was more concerned about the phone call at that hour or the fact that he saw the lights as well. Yes! I scored one point for myself. Either they were real or we were both crazy. No matter which, I was not alone.

One day I had to go downstairs in the hospital for a procedure. While waiting in the room and as they were beginning to administer anesthesia, *I Can Only Imagine* by MercyMe began playing on the radio. It was very eerie and yet peaceful feeling at the same time. When I woke up in the recovery room, I was relieved in some respects and yet disappointed in others. It most certainly changed my perspective on the way that I had been living. It was as though I had been given another chance: to see all that I had been taken for granted and what truly mattered.

My depth perception was off so I had difficulty even feeding myself. There is a lot to be said for missing your mouth with a spoon full of food and having to wear a bib when just three months ago I could eat anything and everything. A fork was completely out of the question. I would have testified that they made the spaces between the prongs of a fork wider because, for the life of me, I couldn't keep food on it. Finger food became a favorite. I'm not talking sandwiches, either. I'm talking about cheez-it crackers! With all of the medication I was on there was a distinct metal taste in my mouth with whatever I ate or drank. Cheese, I found out, would cut that taste. Certainly not the best choice of foods for my kidneys, but they tasted wonderful any time of the day!

On June 29th, the afternoon before I was supposed to be discharged it was just my father and me in the room. If I was going to survive at home Dad and I needed to be able to work together to get what I needed done. Lying in the hospital bed I realized that I needed to go to the bathroom. I had been on bed rest for thirty days because of the blood clot and infection. Even more unsteady on my feet than usual, a bedside commode was placed literally a foot from the edge of my bed. How hard could this be? Sit up, have help standing by the edge of my bed, slowly pivot one-hundred and eighty degrees and sit down.

It was in that brief moment that my father and I realized what we were up against. On my way back to bed, my legs gave out and I hit the floor of my hospital room hard. Bewildered on why it had occurred I just looked up at Dad, helpless and not knowing really what to do next. I did not have the strength to even bring myself to my knees with the help of the bedrail. My father tried his best to lift me. It took all of his strength as well as mine and we did not make much progress. Just shy of one hundred and eighty pounds of dead weight, this was no small task.

Even more than the fact I had to get up off the floor, we were afraid of being caught by one of the nurses or doctors. The event certainly would have bought me a few more days surrounded by the same white walls and they quickly felt as though they were closing in around me. If that had been the case, the staff would either have to place heavy padding on those walls or give me some serious medications. I had lost it being in for so long. By the grace of God, with the help of Dad and after about ten minutes of trying, I finally got back onto my bed. It had not been three minutes and in walks my nurse. I was exhausted from the ordeal but just smiled at the relief of her not walking in sooner. When she left the room Dad and I just laughed out loud and realized we had to be even more cautious with every step that I was to take.

Because my mediport was continuously accessed and my high risk of infection, I was unable to shower. Not enough sponge baths in the world made me feel clean. It had already been two and a half weeks and now they were telling me it would be another six weeks because I had to complete treatment.

I was discharged the evening of Saturday, June 30th with pure determination. It was the last Saturday of June and I was supposed to be healthy, seventeen hundred miles away in Windham, Maine at a lobster bake with family and friends. With little strength and having my father's assistance to walk, I decided on Red Lobster for dinner. I might not have been in Maine but I for sure was going to have the same dinner as them.

At the restaurant I was faced with the choice of going up the ramp or attempting the step along the edge of the sidewalk. Flat surfaces were difficult enough and I could not have even told you the last time stairs were attempted so Dad and I stuck with the ramp. I was almost two-thirds of the way up when my knees buckled. My father caught me so I did not hit the cement but hollered for help because he could not lift me up from the stooped position I had ended in. A passer-by helped me up and that poor gentleman I clung to for dear life until I was stable on my feet again. The manager came out to assist me to our table. When finished, he took us out the side emergency exit that had no ramp or step. That night I ended up sleeping in the recliner in the living room. I could not make it up the stairs to my room and my bed had yet to be setup where I could go.

Home health care arrived the following day and showed my mother, who had absolutely no medical background, how to administer the treatments *once*. I guess she was supposed to be an expert after that. My father, who also had no medical experience, happened to be working that day so when my infusion finished the nurse looked at me and said "You can talk your Dad through this, right? We will come once a week to change the needle." Thank God I had a nursing background! Yeah, sure, no problem. What were these people thinking? The one with the brain infection and the one that needed these medications is supposed to teach others how to make sure they administer them to her correctly? I was on four to six infusions or antibiotics per day, around the clock, for eight weeks. Thank God for my parents because I think I slept through half of them and there was nobody else to take care of me.

Expanding on the concept of cheez-it crackers, I came to discover that I could taste the cheese in macaroni and cheese and the sauce mix used with hamburger helper lasagna. I also ate a great deal of watermelon, had a peanut butter and jelly phase and mint chocolate chip ice cream because it just tasted good. I would not recommend this diet to anyone; however, in the moment it was the best thing in the world!

Being on high doses of prednisone also increased my appetite. There were days when I would literally munch on food from the time I woke up until the time I went to sleep. It was incredible! Mom was staying home with me at the time due to the intravenous infusions. She ran between the kitchen and the living room, where I was, with snacks more times in a twenty-four hour period than I could ever imagine. I believe she lost all the weight I was gaining.

It was during one of my trips to the emergency room that my folks were *venting* about the craziness of the inconsistency of the flow meters on the intravenous tubing. The fact that home health only came once a week did not provide the opportunity for questions to be answered in a timely fashion. The nurse that was working with me that evening told them that in order to calculate the flow rate per minute, count the number of drips per fifteen seconds and multiply by four. Certainly easier than trying to watch and count the drips for a complete minute and it was so simple we could not even think of it on our own.

MRIs became so frequent that they turned into a game for me when I felt well enough. I would be lying still trying to determine what noise pattern the machine would make next. I had a point system for if I got the answer right or not. I didn't do very well and usually lost count before the test was over but it kept me occupied. There were also colorful plastic window stickers of fish that I could see while having my MRI. At the worst of it, I know for certain those fish were moving during my test! It was also those times when I would lay there, trying to be still, and tears were streaming down my face because the headaches became so intense from the pounding of the machine.

I know that throughout my time being diagnosed with lupus, my time with the brain infection has been the most challenging, uncertain, and overwhelming. It was also some of my darkest days. That was not living. I became totally dependent again. I could not stand up on my own. For a time being I could not even sit up on my own. I became dependent on using a bedpan and ladies; I can tell you that there is no worse feeling than having to use one of those things for #2 when only your father is home! I thought I would rather die!

~ Raw ~

Like the peeling of dry skin,
each flake brings a new emotion.
Layers of an onion being sliced,
one by one,
to expose the true core within.
A loss of privacy.

Not having the strength
to simply roll yourself over.
Learning how to walk again
one slow step at a time.
Taking the falls as they come.
A loss of dignity.

Like the rising of the tide
the world is crashing in.
Every move monitored,
words whispered,
another storm is brewing.
A loss of independence.

Not being able to prepare a meal,
get out of bed,
stand,
even hang out with friends.
A loss of pride.

Losing privacy,
dignity,
independence
and pride.
As each layer brings you
a step closer
to raw.

~ *The Dream* ~

This dream occurred only twice and was during the most challenging times with the brain infection. It was not one that overly concerned me at the moment, possibly because I felt so miserable, but there is definitely something to be said for envisioning and planning your own funeral. Even an hour of thinking provided a new perspective and insight on the life that I had.

I woke up startled at the intense visions that had just played out in my mind and reached for a notebook. I was to be cremated and my only flowers were to be a single yellow rose. In lieu of flowers, I wanted a fund established at St. Jude Children's Research Hospital in Memphis, Tennessee to assist patients and families in need. The songs to be played were *She's a Butterfly* by Martina McBride, *I Did It My Way* by Frank Sinatra, *I'll Fly Away* by Jars of Clay, and *Praise You in This Storm* by Casting Crowns. In no particular order, the scripture that I wanted included were Ephesians 2: 8 - 10, John 3:16, John 14: 1-6, and the 23rd Psalm. Messages that have certainly made a difference in my outlook throughout this journey and that you may find and read in *Scripture Reference* directly after the last chapter, *Final Thoughts,* of this book.

I didn't worry about where to be buried. I wanted my ashes tossed into the ocean with the wind so that my free spirit could indeed travel the world to see all the places that I still hoped to visit. I had a list of pros and cons for each choice I made including, of course, the expense I would be leaving behind. I wanted it to be a celebration of my life and not a focus on all I had allowed the disease to make me become.

When alone in the house for the first time since the dream, I reached for the phone and called Kennedy. Knowing each other our entire lives and certainly my best friend, I needed to talk. I needed someone to know what my plans were *just in case* and someone who would be able to later relay the information. Honestly, I did not know how to even begin to tell my parents this information. I guess they will read it here and I hope that they do so knowing, with confidence that I have moved forward.

It took some time for me to realize that I was allowing lupus to control my life. What I could no longer do, what I could no longer eat, and what I could no longer become. It was in the midst of my self-talk and self-pity that I realized I did not want to become a statistic: I wanted to prove everyone wrong and become a survivor.

~ *Sunset* ~

Growing up there was always one place where I was certain to find peace and understanding: down by the shoreline. It was no wonder, after I had been in the house for weeks, my father had the idea to take me to watch sunset down to Pass-A-Grille and with any luck brighten my spirits. What could possibly be better than hearing the waves crash against the shore while a skyline of purple and orange hues illuminated the background?

On a mid-summer evening I slowly made my way to the car, excited at the very thought of getting out not to mention going to one of my favorite places! For some unknown reason I never comprehended the full extent of what this journey would entail. At this point in time I was still very unsteady on my feet, trying to recover from the brain infection, and believing in my heart I was going to have a blast at the beach. Reality quickly brought my thoughts to a halt.

Upon arriving at Pass-A-Grille I slowly and carefully made my way to the back of the car where Dad was waiting with my wheelchair. At that moment I was struck with the realization that I was not there for a typical trip to watch sunset. My feet would not touch the warm sand, I would not feel the grains between my toes and the waves would not be slapping against my ankles as I walked along the water's edge.

We crossed the street, went up the ramp and passed the snack bar to the edge of the cement landing. This was as close as I was getting. My wheelchair was not some magic, all-terrain vehicle that could plow through the sand to get to where I wanted to be. As I looked out across the water, with my folks on either side of me, the tears silently and steadily began flowing down my face. They watched me with a look as though they were not only concerned but confused as well. From their expressions I could tell the questions running through their minds. *Was she hurt or in pain? How could she love the beach so much and be sitting here in tears? I thought this was supposed to cheer her up not make her cry?* The only response that I was able to give was that I wanted to be left alone for a few minutes. Without questioning, they both got up and went for a walk. They walked down onto the sand where I longed to be.

In my mind I could only envision a scene from the movie *City of Angels* where all of the angels wore their black trench coats and were standing along the shore. They could feel the wind against their face, an unwavering sense of contentment and freedom, a love for life itself. I wanted that feeling. Lord knows, more than anything I wanted that feeling at that exact moment. Instead I sat in my chair, tears flowing even heavier now because I was alone and with each passing moment I was becoming more determined to walk again. It was a release of all of the emotions and frustration I had bottled up within me so as not to upset others. I knew at that moment there would be a day when I would stand on the shore and feel the wind against my face again and the waves against my ankles. A time when I would feel that freedom and peace, a love for life greater than anything I had felt before because I was no longer taking it for granted. I became determined that I would see that day again and cherish the memories even more than the thought itself.

43 MOVING FORWARD

~ *Making Progress* ~

During one of my admissions my father was going to stop by and visit after he finished work for the day. Having not eaten all day mother had the great idea of going to Subway to get him a sandwich for when he got there. The only thing she had to do was go out of the hospital driveway and turn right, as if she was headed back to our house, and she would pass it.

Not long after she left I received a phone call. The first words she said to me were: "I'm lost." How did it happen that you went out of the driveway, turned right and got lost finding Subway restaurant? There had been an accident at the next intersection and she had to take a detour. The description I received was that she was by the airport. I didn't think she had enough time to make it to Tampa. I asked her if it was Clearwater/St. Petersburg. She didn't know the answer; it was just an airport down by the water.

Through randomly driving around she was able to tell me that she was by a yacht club. Sweet! I now have some idea where you are in St. Petersburg! I talked her back to Central Avenue, which she was familiar with, and brought her down by Tropicana Field where the Tampa Bay Rays play baseball. By the time that she got back to the intersection, where she had started out, the accident was cleared up. I told her not to bother and just come back to the hospital...she went to Subway anyway because she now knew where she was and knew how to get to where she wanted to be.

I mention this because it was one of the funniest moments of my time in the hospital. I could not wait to tell my father that she had called the kid in the hospital, with the brain infection, to ask directions from somewhere where she didn't know to somewhere that she just wanted to get a sandwich. She told me that I did not have to let Dad know what she had done; however, that was the highlight of my week. I believe it was the first words I spoke when he walked through the door that evening. She can even laugh about it now; however, it was not nearly as comical for her that first night.

There was one afternoon while I was home alone I wormed my way to the edge of the bed and was able to sit up. I took the palms of my hand and went to press them down into the mattress so I was more stable. When I pushed down with my legs as well, I stood up on my own! This was the first time in about six weeks that I had actually stood up without someone else assisting me. It literally scared me so much, with the feeling like I was going to fall, that I sat back down. A minute later I thought that was pretty neat and tried it again.

Mom came into the house first and I impatiently waited for my father to return from work. When we were sitting in the living room that evening I discreetly worked my way to the edge of the bed, sat up and then slowly stood and said: "Hey, check it out!" with a big grin on my face. Every little progress was celebrated as a major milestone in our world at the time. They eventually found out I had been practicing all afternoon. Within a couple weeks, I was able to wobble across the floor in some strange form of walking independently.

There was one point in July when I went into the MRI room and I knew for certain that I had to be doing better. Two of the window stickers were sea horses. It blew me away. I had been going there for two months getting repeat MRIs and never once did I know that those two little pink blurs I had seen while lying in the machine could have been sea horses!

After the antibiotic treatment, when I was able to shower that presented its own challenges. First of all, I had to learn to do stairs again. I found that it was easier for me to go outside and around to the main door of the house because it had a railing. I would literally hold on and put one foot on the step. My weight would then shift so that I was leaning over the railing, pressing down, and with enough momentum was able to get my second foot up. Luckily there were only two steps from the ground into the house and that the railing was able to hold my weight.

Once I got to the main level and down the hallway, I could not lift my leg up over the tub to get it into the shower. Whenever I did want to shower, which was quite frequently those first few days, the glass doors had to be taken off the tub/shower. Then a scatter rug went into the tub before the dining room chair so the chair would not slide. By sitting in the chair, I could literally lift one leg at a time into the bathtub. A removable shower head was a wonderful invention!

~ *One Step at a Time* ~

It went painfully up and to the left
before returning to a normal position.
The rest of my weight
hung like a rag doll
over the railing
in hopes of maintaining
balance and stability.

Catching my breath
after the workout
just completed,
I gently slide
my other leg
up the carpeted side
with hope
it makes it past the little lip
at the top on the first try.
Not doing this once,
but twice.

Energy expenditure -
the things we take for granted.

Open the door,
let me in,
this victory is mine.
I made it
to the main level of the house
one step at a time.

MOVING FORWARD

~ I'm Going Home ~

Victory was mine! The last MRI that I had showed no lesions in the brain. Antibiotics had finally worked and there was only one thing on my mind that I wanted to do: go home to Maine and see my family and friends that had encouraged me every step of the way and had not seen me since I moved to Florida almost a year ago.

Looking at my schedule full of doctor's appointments and blood work it was nearly impossible to find a time suitable for a vacation that was seventeen hundred miles away. That was not even considering the fact that I was still very unsteady on my feet, could not walk up stairs on my own and would definitely have to fly instead of ride in a car for that distance. Hard telling everything that I would have to pack to survive a week away from home. Can you even take that many medications on a plane now? Lord knows with the amount of Lasix I was taking there was absolutely no way I could be too far away from, shall I say, modern conveniences. My mind kept racing with questions and everything that it would entail to pull off a trip like this and yet, I was determined.

Since being diagnosed with the brain infection, one thing kept coming to mind: I wanted to see my brother, Joe, and I could not figure out why he wasn't here. The thought of him working five or more days a week was not conducive to the schedule of his sister which included working on gaining my strength but mostly laying in bed staring off into space and having all day and night to mull through my own thoughts. Looking back, I can honestly say that the mass quantity of time I spent mulling through my own thoughts really was *not* therapeutic.

It was by a combination of many phone calls, rescheduling appointments, and having all doctors clear me that one entire week became available. My folks realized how much I wanted this and they were anxious to get back home as well and see everyone. I believed that more than anything, I was looking forward to a week away from all that my life had become. For an entire week I did not have to see a doctor, I did not have to get stuck with a needle for some blood work or intravenous infusion, and I did not have to lie on some stretcher for a medical procedure deemed necessary due to my condition. For one entire week I would be free from it all, free from what my life had become.

The trip home was interesting to say the least. Going through the airport I felt degraded by others. Seriously, who sees a twenty-nine year old woman cruising around in a wheelchair at the airport with a face and body like a very full chipmunk due to prednisone? By that point in time I had already gained about fifty pounds due to my condition and medications. I felt like it would have been easier to roll but God knows I wouldn't have been able to stand on my own after I stopped! Because of my weakened immune system I also had to wear a mask in public. The entire flight and ride around the airport I had a mask covering half my face. I knew people around me believed I should just get up and walk like the rest of them. What was wrong with me that I had to board the plane before everyone else and then be the last one off so I could get into a wheelchair and be escorted wherever I went?

Little did I comprehend the lasting impression I would be leaving on my brother and best friend who met me in Portland, Maine at the airport when I arrived. The initial look on their faces told it all. I looked like crap and after a day of travel it seriously must have been worse. I was literally the last one off the plane, my father pushing the wheelchair, and the only distinguishing part of me was my blue eyes sparkling with relief that the day was almost over.

Because of my limited abilities as well as a strong desire to see practically everyone I knew back home within a week, a party was scheduled at our summer camp for the Saturday we would be home. It was three days after we arrived so that I would have time to recuperate from the plane ride and a few days before having to make the trip back. I was amazed and overwhelmed with the number of people that saved the date, with such short notice, just to come visit with my folks and me. Because I could not do stairs without assistance, I spent my day on the deck of the camp and everyone had to come to me.

With help, I had posters made of a time line for what I had been through, what I was thankful for as well as lupus facts and diagnostic criteria. That was one of the best things I did for that day because not only did people just stand there in amazement but it also seriously cut back on the repetitive questions. Even one of my friends would chime in and respond with 'go read the posters' when questions came up. It became a game for the two of us by the end of it, sort of like a quiz to see who had actually read them before coming to see me.

There were mixed reactions from people that saw me while I was home. There were a few that did not talk with me but spoke to Mom and Dad about me. Some turned away in tears because yes, I looked that different from how they had known me a year prior. Others just acted like they normally would around me and then there were the chosen few that never left my side the entire time they were visiting. It was interesting that many took on that parent role of asking me if I was alright and if there was anything they could do for me. I went from being confined in the living room with two parents to being on the deck at camp with about thirty. Every minute of it was worth it because these were my true friends and family. They were standing beside me, seeing me at some of my worst moments and loving me anyway.

Joe bought dinner for me one night. As a special treat he came back from town with lobsters. Even I was amazed at how quickly the first one disappeared from my plate. I had nobody to blame but myself and in total I ate three that night and completely worried my folks that I was going to be sick. They tasted delicious and for as much as I ate I was even surprised I did not so much as get a stomachache from it. A rare, thoughtful treat that came in part of my brother's way for showing how much he cared and how much he was glad to have me home, even for a week.

One of the hardest things for me to realize while I was there was that I could not walk down and sit by the edge of the lake. Being unsteady was not compatible with the unevenness of the ground down by the water. If I fell, it would have been overwhelmingly difficult to get back onto my feet. It reminded me of sunset and how determined I was to get by the shoreline again. Progress had already been made because I could walk, okay wobble, short distances. Soon I would feel that contentment, freedom and love for life on my own once more.

As usual, a week of vacation went by way too fast. I could tell it had been a great week because it would take about another week to get caught up on all the rest I had missed while back home. The flight back was about as interesting as the flight there. I arrived safe and exhausted back in Florida and my bed in the living room never looked so good. I just wanted and needed to crash but every moment away had been worth it and exceeded the expectations even my dreams had held.

~ One Day at a Time ~

As much as I wanted to push myself harder and harder to get well again, there were constant little reminders to take things one day at a time.

Sometime during one of my admissions after the brain infection and before I had actually regained a great deal of strength I happened to fall. It was late at night and I had pressed the button to notify the nurse that I needed some help. Being in nursing at one point myself, after about ten minutes of waiting, I shut the call light off and decided I would get up and venture to use the bathroom by myself. Of course, I had an IV pole to tote along with me but I figured it would help steady me. Unfortunately, I could not reach over to my top drawer where my socks were. No big deal, I have walked barefoot hundreds of times. I made it there fine but on my way back I had to reach across the back of my bed and plug the IV pump in so it would not run the battery down. Little was I expecting to bump into the corner of the wheel and it would be enough to knock me off balance and I hit the floor.

My dilemma then became either to shout for the nurse to come pick me up off the floor, in which case she didn't know I was up and I didn't have socks on, or to do whatever I had to in order to get back into bed before being caught. I opted for the second choice! After about ten minutes of struggling and not being able to support my own weight on my knees I used the bedrail and reached across the mattress to literally haul myself up onto the bed. As exhausted as I was from the exertion I also realized I had to boost myself up because I was so close to the foot of the bed I couldn't even stretch out. I was proud of my independent accomplishment and was laughing as I also realized that this technique could be used for future reference in case I ever found myself in that situation again…which I did, after I returned home and fell on our living room floor.

During the summer of 2008, while in Maine, I acquired shingles on my lower back. At that time, I was seeing a doctor at the Alfond Center in Augusta for treatment. His response was *it is shingles* and gave me a prescription to have filled. Unfortunately, my pharmacy was in Florida and Maine did not accept my insurance. By the time the medication arrived it was of little help. The area only got worse and the doctor did not care to look at it again because he knew what it was. One night, while still in Maine, I was running a low-grade fever and had an interesting dream of an armadillo chasing me and then attacking. I told my folks that it had to be true because I had the marking to prove it: where the shingles and raw skin was on my lower back.

Once I returned to Florida, to my regular doctors the beginning of September, many layers of skin were gone covering an area of about three inches by two inches. It was literally a dwelling at the base of my back. I ended up having to be sent to the wound care center for debridement of the area and a special ointment applied in order for it to heal.

In January 2009, I was admitted to the hospital with headaches again. A battery of tests were completed and it was determined that I had migraines. Throughout my time there I was overdosed on barbiturates and, at one point, passed out on the floor and woke up to a team surrounding me because a code had been called. I wasn't myself. I would sit in a chair and just rock back and forth. I did not want anyone to touch me, talk with me or even look at me. While I was still in the hospital, I became paranoid that others were watching me and somehow out to get me. I wanted to be left completely alone. I knew I was not myself and it was affecting every aspect of my life when a friend called and asked: 'are you over-emotional lately or is something else going on with you?' I cannot even tell you how many messages I had left for him. The more messages he received the crazier they sounded.

53 MOVING FORWARD

My last hospital admission was definitely my shortest stay yet was related to chest pain and difficulty breathing. I went through a battery of tests in the emergency room, received three nitroglycerine tablets and then was brought upstairs and admitted to a private room. The nitroglycerine tablets did ease the chest pain but it also caused a horrific headache! After fifteen hours and seeing a few different doctors I was told that nothing was wrong and I could either hang out for the night on observation or go home to my own bed. I left and came home realizing there was nothing they were going to do for me if I stayed and I could at least get a better night sleep at home in my own bed.

One of the most interesting aspects of this journey has been how I viewed things as a patient versus how I viewed them when I was the nurse. Honestly, there were times that I would not have seen anyone for hours at a time if my folks were not with me in the hospital. The staff would be in to take my vital signs, drop off meals and give me medication. Please don't take this wrong. Not every nurse was like this but I have certainly met a lot of them. I remember getting so frustrated at night because it seemed the later it got the louder it was in the hallway. I was usually close by the nurse's station as well, which didn't help the situation. The sounds of the hole puncher, stapler and, most of all, ring binders at night was enough to drive me crazy. It was also interesting to see the nurses that seemed to use my bed and table for the chart, medication packaging, IV flush wrappers, alcohol swabs, etc. There were times when I felt like the Peanuts character Pig Pen and there was this little cloud of dust that followed me wherever I went. I realized it was different working with pediatrics but I would lay there and seriously hope that some of the things that were happening were not how I treated the children and their families.

I don't know where life is headed or how long I am going to be here. What I have learned is to enjoy the moment. Don't live in the past and don't live for the future, live in the moment.

Do not dwell upon what you can no longer do or how you no longer look, be thankful for the gift of today and all the little blessings that come with it.

~ *A Taste of Freedom* ~

September 4, 2008 I woke up early and asked my parents what they thought about me going to Daytona for the night after I had blood work later that morning. Neither one of them were impressed with the idea, let alone the thought of me driving three plus hours on my own to get there. Ultimately, they told me their thoughts and said that it was my decision. By one o'clock that afternoon my decision was the complete and total opposite of their thoughts. I was going...more than anything; I was going alone and I was going to prove a point.

I needed to know that after everything I had been through I was not totally dependent. I needed to know that I could actually go somewhere if I wanted to, in my car and with my own free will. I needed to know that I could get in the car and just take off to see a friend. I needed them to know that I was not so fragile and I would not break if I got out for the day. This was the furthest away from home I had been on my own since moving back in with my folks in December 2006. It was also the longest period of time I had been away unless, of course, you count hospital admissions...which I try not to. I felt like a kid again, so excited to be heading out on another great adventure, so excited for that taste of freedom.

One of my friends whom I had met on the second road trip to Daytona back when I first moved to Florida was working at Volusia mall that evening. He didn't know I could drive across the state let alone that I was going just to see him. The ride over was exhilarating! The radio was on, the windows were down and, for once in a very long time, I was going somewhere not as a passenger.

By this point I had been off prednisone for six months and looked closer to my normal self that he was accustom to seeing. When I arrived at the mall I went to walk into the store and he was with a customer. I caught his eye and made a ninety-degree turn for the bench with a big grin on my face. I didn't know if he recognized me but I knew I couldn't just walk in while he was busy. So I waited.

He had recognized me immediately and it was so good to see each other again. One thing that he did comment about struck me instantly. He had not seen me since before I was diagnosed and I refused to send him pictures of my awful looking stages with prednisone and the brain infection, etc. He told me that when he saw me again he did not know if he was going to have to fight back tears...but that I looked good. I looked him in the eyes and said, "If that had been the case, I wouldn't have come". As much as he encouraged, supported me and showed me strength, never once did I want him to see me sick. He is the one that would tell me that the experience would make me stronger and that I needed to keep moving forward. His comment made me realize an entirely different perspective. Even when I loathed my appearance, and God knows there was quite a while with that thought, I didn't stop and think about how others would react to seeing me. I realized when I went home to Maine it was a shock for most people but I never questioned their thoughts and feelings behind the mixed reactions.

That night we rented a movie, had some popcorn, shared some white zinfandel wine and just had the opportunity to talk face to face again and hang out together after so long. It was so good to see him again. The following morning I was the one to wake up with mixed emotions. I was so grateful for the time that I had been there but upset with the fact that I had to leave so soon. I drove back in a steady rain from the outskirts of a tropical development. For twenty-four hours I was free. I was free to relax and truly be myself. I was free from all that my life had become and back close to living the life that I had known and lost. I loved every minute of it and am so thankful for the time we shared!

MOVING FORWARD

~ The Bionic Woman ~

A major yearly event in Plant City, Florida is the Strawberry Festival. I love to attend and was looking forward again to the entertainment, food and festivities surrounding the event.

The first year I was in Florida and attended, it was a few weeks after I was diagnosed with lupus. The day after I went, I was readmitted to the hospital due to complications with my kidney function. The day before I planned on attending the following year, I had an appointment with my doctors in Gainesville. My right hip had been bothering me to the point that it was painful to walk and could not even lie on that side while trying to sleep. While speaking with my doctors, it was determined that I would receive a cortisone shot to see if that would alleviate some discomfort. That night, it felt great!

The following day I got up excited and ready to go. We had tickets to see the afternoon headline entertainment, Crystal Gale, took in every Vocal Trash performance we could and I ate everything I probably shouldn't have yet it was so good. By early afternoon my hip was starting to bother again and I figured it was because of the extensive activity I had that morning. It had been a long time since I had done that much walking in one day. My folks and I went to the afternoon show and part way through it I could not even sit still in the chair. I couldn't get comfortable sitting, standing or even trying to walk around on the outside of the rows of chairs. I was in so much pain that I felt nauseous. I wanted to ask if anyone had some cortisone. It seemed to work twenty four hours ago and right then I was willing to try anything.

We stayed for the remainder of the show and then were going to leave the festival. I walked slowly and staggering back towards the exit and about halfway there had literally gone as far as I could and collapsed onto one of the picnic table benches. Much to my dismay, my father went to get a wheelchair to bring me the rest of the way to the car. I couldn't even stand on my right leg. Kindly enough, which was not what I thought at the moment, there was not a wheelchair available so the rescue team came to pick me up in their vehicle and take me to the car. Nothing like a little white paddy wagon to carry me away and off the festival grounds. If looks could have killed my father would have been the one to drop there and need a ride! They were even kind enough to run the siren for me. I can laugh about it now but I certainly was not laughing in the moment. If I hadn't been in so much pain I probably would have waved at the people we were passing, like a queen, as though I was part of a parade.

From the festival I went straight to the hospital emergency room in St. Petersburg. Unfortunately, the staff did not feel as thought it was an *emergency*. They sat me in a wheelchair and I literally sat and was never taken out back to be seen by a doctor for over five hours. Of course, the staff would not give me anything for pain because I had not seen the doctor yet and they were unsure what would be done for testing.

When x-rays showed that I had avascular necrosis of the ball joint for my hip it was determined that I was going to be admitted. Another hurdle to cross was finding a bed available. The hospital was full and I ended up spending the night in the emergency room. I had arrived at 6:45pm and was never taken upstairs to a room until 10:15 the following morning!

The deterioration had been caused by long term high doses of prednisone. My options now were to be weaned completely off steroids and have a total hip replacement. Before a replacement could take place, fluid needed to be drawn out of the right hip to make sure that there was no infection and I was on bed rest until doctors could figure out what to do with me.

When left alone, I called a friend. I needed to laugh, I needed a friendly voice and I needed to occupy my mind with thoughts other than another hospital admission. We spoke of fitting in a little too well with the retirement community, I could have races with a walker as part of my rehabilitation and the possibility of going dancing. Of course, with a bum hip it would make dancing so much more interesting! I would have to be careful doing the Hokey Pokey because putting my right hip either in or out could be detrimental and then eventually comical, let alone the thought of shaking it all about or turning myself around. I needed the laughter, the brighter outlook and the comforting voice of a friend.

Physical therapy came in to work with me and was teaching me how to use a walker prior to surgery. With the help of the walker I made it a step or two beyond the end of my bed. No great adventure but further than I had walked in a few days. Morphine was administered quite regularly and most of the time it didn't matter to me if it was daylight or dark. At times, I was lucky to know the difference.

Six days after I arrived in the emergency room I had a right total hip replacement and four days following that I was released to go home. I would have a home health nurse come in and check the wound and remove the staples about a week and a half post-surgery.

There was some discussion about me being transferred to a rehabilitation facility following surgery to work with physical therapy. My insurance, at the time, would not pay for home health as well as a physical therapist to come to the house. I was determined to make it on my own at home.

For a while there would be no weight-bearing at all and then I would gradually increase after that from just toe touching to some weight bearing and eventually full weight bearing. That schedule really did not work for me and so I worked a little harder and a little longer each day, did physical therapy on my own and was actually full weight bearing four week post operation. I made my father carry my walker out of the doctor's office. I was done with it! I could do stairs with the assistance of a railing, transfer in and out of the car, and stand up long enough to cook without any discomfort.

To occupy my time while I was home lying around, my brother sent me a Wii game system. Nothing was more comical than the look on my surgeon's face when I told him that within a week and a half after surgery I took up bowling and tennis! I got great pleasure from making him wonder for a few seconds before actually telling him it was on the Wii and I could do it lying down without weight bearing.

A great disappointment, okay not that great in the grand scheme of things but regardless, occurred on May 29, 2008 when I went through airport security on a trip back to Maine and the stainless steel did not set the alarm off. I was so excited and had my card ready to show the airport attendants and nothing happened. Mom called me nuts for even wanting it to go off. I just thought it would be neat and was disappointed. I think it was the first thing I told my brother after saying hello when he picked me up at the airport in Portland. The alarm didn't go off but at least I was not being wheeled around the airport or the last one off the plane this year!

September 16, 2008, I went back to the hospital and had a left total hip replacement. My left hip was more deteriorated than the right and they ended up taking more bone and replacing it with more stainless steel. I lost more blood with this operation and needed five pints transfused before being discharged a week following surgery. Even though this replacement bothered more than the first, I pushed myself to be full weight bearing a little sooner. I had too much to do to be down for a month. Two and a half weeks after this surgery I was walking without assistance. I would not recommend being up and on your own that quickly now; however, in the moment, it felt as though I had used the walker for months.

Five and a half weeks following my second hip replacement there was a seafood festival down to John's Pass in

Madeira Beach. My father was working there and I decided, during some obviously lack of common sense moment, it would be a great idea to walk down there and visit as well as go to the festival. I started walking and knew that once I got to the Madeira Beach elementary school I could take a free shuttle the remainder of the way. Little did I calculate that it was 3.8 miles just to get to the school.

The adventure started off great. I crossed two busy roads with six lanes of traffic each and slowly made my way towards the beach. Not really keeping in mind that I was not supposed to be in the sun, I left early afternoon with a hat, a couple bottles of water, and some sun screen on. Every bus stop had a bench and I think that I sat to rest on every one of them that day! I never thought I would make it to the school let alone John's Pass.

By the time that my mother called during her break at work I had just reached the elementary school. I was physically exhausted. She about lost it when I told her where I was. Just boarding the shuttle for the second round of my trip. I was never so glad to get to John's Pass and my father was never more concerned to see me and wondered how on earth I had gotten there. My response: the first mode of transportation invented...my own two feet! I was completely worn out by the time I made it to the festival, to the point that I could not even walk around and enjoy it. I sat in my car, which my father had taken to work, with the air conditioner on and took a nap. No matter, it was a priceless accomplishment with my two stainless steel hips. By accomplishing that, I realized I could go anywhere.

~ *Gulfcoast Oncology* ~

    The staff and patients at Gulfcoast Oncology have become my extended family. These are the people that saw me through every step of the way. The good, the bad, most certainly the ugly and no matter what met me with a smile and words of encouragement and support.
    I visited the unit at least every week, sometimes more frequently around hospital admissions. Here, they took care of everything from blood work to shots for helping bring up my blood counts to chemotherapy infusions to happy meals (minus the toy) of fluid when I would get dehydrated and definitely inspirations as well as contributing to this wacky sense of humor I now carry around with me. No matter when I went in, and it still continues to this day, it is like picking up with a friend you haven't seen in a while, right where you left off the last time you were together.
    This unit is a place where one can go and be accepted...no matter what changes your system or physical appearance is dealing with. Everyone understands what you are going though, is willing to help you through it and we have a lot of fun together along the journey.
    Dr. Dolan is the most patient, kind and understanding person I have found within this profession. Never have I seen her without a smile or being upbeat. She provided us with hope when options were running low and encouragement when things were going rough. She kept in close contact with other doctors on the team and discussed all ideas and options with us before any final decision was made. Thank God we met her on this journey.
    After I first started going into Gulfcoast, my mother would call the office and usually get Doris on the phone. She knew us immediately and would do whatever was needed: an appointment, a visit to the doctor or even call ahead for us if we were headed into the emergency room. Kim has now taken on the job, actually there are two Kims that work in the main office and they both

know me when I call. My phone calls are primarily to ask for blood work results at this point; however, no matter who I am speaking with, they always ask how I am really doing, not just if I am doing okay.

Being on a regular schedule, I would usually see the same people week after week and we would get joking around. When one of us would have our port accessed or an IV started, someone else would yell 'ouch' for them across the room. The day of my thirtieth birthday, I was receiving a four hour infusion. It was then that I took a little cocktail umbrella in with me and put it slightly into one of the ports in the IV line between the machine and myself. We joked that it was the only cocktail I had been allowed to have, a martini minus the olive because it would get stuck in the tubing. We would ask for frequent flyer miles so as soon as treatment was over we could bust out of there, travel the world and get back to living. Don't worry, we would send a postcard. Each week I would try to wear a different t-shirt with a new and crazy saying on it to either make others laugh or read it and ponder. For a few weeks we would take turns on who was going to bring the snacks because sometime between the intravenous steroids and Benadryl we were sure to get the munchies.

On days of my infusions, Dad would usually go with me and we would bring the cribbage board. Four hours worth of fun led to some very interesting games where we would lose track of counting, how many times we had been around the board because it felt like at least a hundred and whose turn it was to deal. To think, I was the only one getting the medicine but it affected both of us!

February 5, 2008 was my last dose of Cytoxan after a six month round of treatment. I went in that day for my infusion as normal but, before I left, the nurses came up with a certificate saying that I had graduated. That round was over and I had to admit that was the best graduation certificate I ever received. Of no others, have I been prouder or had a more eventful journey achieving it.

The nurses in this office have a true bond, one that shows in all they do. They join in when you are having fun and try to boost your spirits when you are down. This is the only place I know of that an entire conversation can consist around Krispy Kreme donuts and peanut butter fudge. They are a team and they work as a team, everyone contributes. They are part of the reason why I am still alive today and why I am able to write this story.

All of this teamwork, all of the doctors and staff as well as the patients must work together to provide this type of welcoming environment. I have seen many different doctors' offices where this environment does not work. At Gulfcoast Oncology, I go in knowing that I am in the best of hands and receiving the greatest of care.

~ *The Research Hospital* ~

First and foremost, thank God for research. The advances in medicine and technology have been overwhelming and a great asset to millions of people.

Along my journey I was referred to two doctors at a research hospital about two and a half hours away. Herein lays the problem. When referred to such a hospital, or doctor, you become at least one of three people:

1) The person enrolled in a research study just wrapping up

2) The person enrolled in a research study just beginning

3) The person enrolled in a research study they are trying to collect data and receive funding for

Every three months, for fifteen minutes, I was seen by these two doctors. After this brief encounter, I walked out with a new treatment plan, different or changed doses in medications, and a greater uncertainty of how my system was going to react. I then traveled back home the two and a half hours, with all changes in place, for my team of doctors to monitor me and deal with any adverse affects that were to take place. They had their work cut out for them.

I have taken Cellcept and Imuran three times each and amazingly enough they still do not work for me. Yet, in the research aspect, I should keep trying. Forget it! This is my body dealing with the side effects and I'm done. This was very frustrating to my doctors because I am steering away from one of the three people in the realm of participating in research and was almost a waste of time and they didn't know what to do with me. The Cellcept caused so many adverse effects, including digestive problems, I could barely function throughout the day and, for me, a week on Imuran led me to renal failure. The doctors tried to convince me it was just a coincidence and had nothing to do with the medication, although it occurred each of the three times.

My doctors finally told me that I needed to decide who was *driving* my course of treatment. Would it be my doctors in St. Petersburg or them in Gainesville? I wanted to ask if they were serious with this question. I see my doctors in St. Petersburg more than once a quarter and they are the ones that have to try and help me when something does go wrong and every time I am admitted to the hospital. Yes, I could travel back and forth to Gainesville more often but why don't we try a little more communication between doctors and see where things go from there?

A great example for lack of communication was the last round of Rituxan I was taking. It was scheduled, in St. Petersburg, as one dose a week for four weeks and then once a month as maintenance. I had one complete dose and the following week went to my appointment in Gainesville and was scheduled for my second dose the following day back in St. Petersburg. After receiving my pre-medications and about one-third of the Rituxan, my doctors in Gainesville had called to stop the infusions for at least two weeks until we could get the results from my blood work back. They were testing my markers to see how active the lupus was at that point in time. I emailed my doctor in Gainesville two weeks later to find out that the test was never done, although it had been requested, and needed to be redone at the lab I go to locally. Hold off on the Rituxan at least until I went back to see them in two and a half months.

There needs to be a better system in place for communication among the team of doctors and everyone needs to be a team player. At times, it gets to the point that everyone is trying to make decisions about what course of treatment should be taken and most of the time they are contradicting each other. Not that either one is necessarily wrong, they are just different. That is when you, as the patient, need to step up and say what you feel is best for you and you alone. Nobody can tell you how you feel or what is exactly going to work for your system. There will be a time when detours will be taken but that is how you learn not to take that path again and explore more options. Don't become a lab rat just for the sake of more studies if it is working against your own system.

I have also learned that a research hospital and staff are not the most receptive people for sharing information with others. Although requested, I never received information from any of my blood tests or urine tests. It was my information; I had a right to see it and yet, never got it. It also took over three weeks of nagging, on my part, to have the results of a kidney biopsy sent to another doctor for evaluation.

~ *Getting By* ~

There are many key moments that helped me to get by the day to day frustration of this journey. Without these moments in time I can honestly say that life would have been a whole lot more difficult. Greatest of all was maintaining a positive outlook. Believe me, not every moment was positive but overall I attempted to look at the brighter side of things.

One of the best gifts we receive in this life is true friendship. These are the people that are not only there for the really great times but, as I have quickly learned, see you through the really hard times. They are the ones that you can call and tell anything to and they listen and accept you. True friends are the individuals who when ask how you are doing really want to know the answer, not just *I'm good*. True friends are the ones who can tell just by the tone of your voice that you called for a specific reason or conversation. Without my friends and family, I would not be alive today. They have been my support system through good and bad alike. Most of my family and friends were still in Maine, seventeen hundred miles away, but were always there when I needed them. What few I had in Florida were the ones that recognized the slightest of accomplishments and reminded me of what progress had been made. If I had lost my family and friends, I would have lost my mind.

Nights were the worst time for me, especially when I was in the hospital. Something about the darkness and loneliness that would settle within me and felt as though it would never go away. Most of my phone calls were made in the evening to attempt to keep my spirits high throughout the night. I carried around a phone card as well as my cell phone in case I needed one of those talks to keep me focused and fighting to get better. I hated the silence and being left with my own thoughts.

69 MOVING FORWARD

When I would get completely frustrated is when I would shut down and not talk. It was in those moments of *don't look at me, don't talk to me and don't touch me* that I could do my greatest reflecting. The realization of where I was compared to where I wanted to be. I'm not talking about where I physically wanted to be because that was always somewhere other than where I was; however, where I wanted to be in life and what I wanted to accomplish before it was over. No matter how much I hated the moment, in the end, I wanted to love life.

Reading Scripture was an important aspect of helping me to get by. It was not my place to understand why this was happening to me rather, what I could learn from it. Certain verses I would try hard to memorize and, even if I forgot, would have them written out and tucked away in a special place. Such verses included James 1: 2 - 4; Philippians 4: 6, 7; Hebrews 4: 14, 15; and Romans 8:28. These verses helped to keep me strong and maintain a brighter outlook. You may find and read these passages in *Scripture Reference* directly after the last chapter, *Final Thoughts*, of this book.

Music was also an important part of my life as well as my recovery. I had always enjoyed an eclectic variety of music to begin with and this journey expanded the horizons even further to help me get by. Not only did it relax me to listen to music, depending on what I was listening to, it could also help encourage me to move. One of the best gifts I received from a friend was an iPod nano. I could take my music anywhere, no matter if to lift my spirits, help me relax or just reflect on the meaning of the songs. There was a point, during *The Storm*, that I could only somewhat freely move the upper half of my body and the lower half was about impossible to move independently. Three songs in particular, all by Barry Manilow, became a wonderful stress reliever for my folks and me. I am not exactly positive how *Mandy*, *Copacabana* and *Looks like We Made It* became a part of our daily routine; however, it was some of the craziest karaoke and antics to accompany them. The harder we laughed the crazier the antics became and the longer it went on. Traveling in the car while listening to these songs always led to an interesting experience! It was during those moments that we could step away from all that life had become and focus on just having fun. On a more serious note, I found great comfort in songs by such artists as Jars of Clay and Mark Schultz.

When I could tolerate sound, television shows such as Montel and 7th Heaven helped pass the time. I was encouraged by the stories that Montel Williams would have on his show as well as his own determination to keep moving forward and coping with multiple sclerosis. I did not want lupus to define me as an individual yet, there were some days, I did not know which direction to take to get well. Sometimes I did not want to move at all and just allow the world to meet me where I was. Even in life's roughest moments there was always a glimmer of hope, something to hold onto and something to believe in. It was a show like Montel's that helped me realize how much I could gain from this experience instead of focusing on all that I had lost.

I avoided mirrors and, for a while, even pictures. I hated my appearance and I did not want to know what I looked like. It was a coping mechanism for getting by because, honestly, if I had taken notice of myself it would have caused greater frustration and depression. I knew what I could physically do and what I wanted to do. Remaining focused on that and not *looking* at all I had lost and was unable to do provided me with the courage to move. I could start from nothing and, with the help of family and friends, could slowly take things one step at a time.

Dr. Manus Praserthdam was one of the first doctors that I met at the time of diagnosis. He would come in, ask questions and then leave only to return a few minutes later with more questions. He kept us informed about what tests were being ordered, why they were ordered and what information he was hoping to find out from them. On February 6, 2007 when I first went into the hospital, he is the one that questioned lupus. Again on the 13th of February when the diagnosis was given, it was he who came in and said 'don't worry, I fix'. He has been an intrinsic part of my folks and me getting by. Dr. Praserthdam informed us that the first year would be the most difficult, there would be more testing, different combinations of medications to see what would work best for my system and we honestly did not know what was ahead of us. When all others had given up hope, he was still saying 'don't worry, I fix'. No matter how bad things seemed, I always believed him and those words. Even when I was diagnosed with the brain infection, he never gave up. It was my rheumatologist that walked away and said nothing more could be done. He came back with a new plan of action from infectious disease and got me back on my feet again.

    When I became ill, I lost all desire to write. Prior to this I had primarily written poetry and it seemed like a memory from another lifetime. My first attempt at creativity, since being diagnosed with lupus, came after my week long trip home in August 2007 after recovering from the brain infection. At that point in time my Uncle was struggling to survive with a brain tumor. We had an unspoken understanding of how things were going, an understanding that others could not quite figure out. The question 'how are you' never had to come up because we already knew the answer. We understood the effects of chemotherapy and the *brain fog* that seemed to accompany it. He would tell me that he admired my strength and called me an inspiration. I gained even more strength from him. His favorite scripture passage, and the one he was teaching his granddaughter, was John 3:16. I wanted to make something special for him that Christmas and decided on a wall hanging made by cross-stitch with this verse. It took me almost until Christmas to complete it, but I was determined. As I was working on each letter and each word I would contemplate the meaning of what I was doing. Was it simply enough to just be doing this for my Uncle of was there something more that I was to learn from this experience? These were not just words I was putting together for a wall hanging but words that came with an overwhelmingly powerful meaning after all I had been through.

    I tried to keep up a strong front, even if I felt like dying on the inside. Nobody wants to be around someone who is depressed or completely frustrated. One of my favorite phrases became *it's all good*. No matter how bad things seemed I kept in mind that it could always be worse. These are the words that helped me to keep my outlook in perspective and to help me get by instead of just going through the motions.

~ *Building a Strong Foundation* ~

After I had *The Dream,* during the roughest trials of my journey, I began to question my own existence. Why was I on earth, what was my purpose for living through everything I had and how could I make a difference with whatever time I had left? Everyone speaks of, and at times even jokes about, a Heaven and Hell but after someone dies it is believed the deceased went to Heaven. Was everyone automatically saved in those final moments, their final breaths, or was there something I was seriously missing? Either way I wanted to know.

I had grown up attending the Catholic Church in Skowhegan, Maine. It was something that we did every week: get up on Sunday, go to church and then go visit my grandparents. Occasionally, we would go on Saturday nights or not at all if there were interfering plans for Sunday. It then got to the point that we went for major holidays, okay Christmas. My sophomore year of high school I started attending church again on a regular basis, as I was to make my confirmation in May. My maternal grandparents were to be my sponsors and, at that point, my grandmother was battling breast cancer. More than anything, I was determined to make my confirmation so she could be there to stand beside me. She passed away less than three months later.

When I left home in the fall of 1996 for college, the first time, I started attending church because I wanted to. It was a choice that I made on my own and the college that I attended had services right on campus every Sunday evening. Within a couple years, I had drifted away again. I had gotten so caught up with living my life, trying to build a future and being independent that I lost my foundation. I felt as though I didn't need help, there was no one thing I was living for and I was doing just fine on my own. Interestingly enough, as I look back at it now, when something went wrong it was 'why did God allow this to happen?' I went to services occasionally but never really seemed to build relationships with those in church around me and never felt as though I was getting out of the sermons what I should be. Reflecting on the service and studying Scripture were two things I was definitely not familiar with nor was it encouraged.

After moving to Florida in 2006 and becoming ill, the thought of attending church was out of the question. I was lucky to get out of the house and, when I did, it was to go to a doctor's appointment or to be readmitted to the hospital for an extended stay. *The Dream* made me realize that I honestly could not look back on my life and discover some great accomplishment, some profound way I had made a difference during my time here or even where I would be going when I died. Heaven and Hell were becoming, in my thoughts and mind, real places and I realized which one I never wanted to be a part of.

Recently having a hip replacement, in March 2008, I was unable to get out and about again. I started listening to the Sunday services of a local church online. I didn't know exactly what I was looking for but I knew there was something missing in my life. I knew that with what I had been through I should not be alive. There were people that had seen me through everything and would tell me I was a miracle. I realized there had to definitely be a *higher power* at work in my life, there was no other way to explain my survival.

It was also about that time I, once again, reached for the phone to call a friend. He was there to listen to me ramble about whatever thoughts came to mind, to answer what questions arose about things that I had heard or read about in Scripture and to explain concepts in terms I could understand. He suggested that I read the Gospel of John, in the New Testament, first to build a foundation before trying to read any other book of the Bible. I had been attempting to read it through from Genesis to Revelation and losing concentration and comprehension quickly. I had a King James Version of the Bible which was very confusing for me to understand the language. It was he who suggested the New King

James Version because it is easier to comprehend and I could better understand things as he explained them if we were looking at the same text. He has been there to discuss everything from specific chapters to a single verse. One of the greatest gifts is that he has been there to accept me as I am. He met me where I was on my journey, stood beside me and helped me to learn and grow from there.

November 16, 2008 and both hip replacements later, I started attending Starkey Road Baptist Church in Seminole, Florida. This is the local church where I had been listening to Pastor Lancaster's services online for months. Not only did I start attending morning service but Sunday school as well. I entered a ten-week New Believer's class and on December 21, 2008 I was baptized. This time as an adult, by my own choosing and with a much greater understanding of why and what I was doing. Every experience, good and bad alike, has helped to make me who I am today. They have all been stepping stones to building my foundation which, I am proud to say, is now stronger than ever.

~ *Final Thoughts* ~

It has been three years since I was diagnosed with lupus. I am often asked where I am at in my treatments, what the prognosis is, what on earth I do with all my *spare time* and what I want to do with my life. Honestly, sometimes the last question makes me want to laugh and sometimes it makes me want to cry.

If anyone had said to me five years ago that this is where I would be today, I would have laughed and called them absolutely crazy. Never did my life plan include living in a retirement community by the age of thirty, being a snowbird, drawing social security, having two stainless steel hips and writing a book about a disease I started off knowing little about. That was not me.

I was the one who loved a challenge; who, after receiving two college degrees, wanted to look into medical school and become a pediatric oncologist; who wanted to travel the world and make a name for myself. I wanted a house and a family. Ultimately, I wanted to work at St. Jude Children's Research Hospital in Memphis, Tennessee. I wanted the experience of a mission trip, not only for the cultural experience but also to assist people in need. I wanted independence and freedom as well as to have every possible adventure I could take in. I wanted the 'perfectionist' quality in all that I attempted and nothing holding me or my dreams back from becoming all that I desired. No matter where my life led, I wanted my work to involve helping others, especially children. Look at me now...

One of my greatest challenges, at this point, is memory loss. There is a great deal of my childhood that I cannot remember. Trips that I know we took as a family, spending time with extended family and even some of the holiday celebrations. Part of my adulthood I recall only through stories friends have told me. Sometimes I can recall the event and sometimes I have no idea what they are talking about. I keep lists for everything to help keep me organized, a calendar that I always have with me and I am very much a fan of speed dial and built in contact lists on cell phones so I do not have to remember phone numbers.

Because of my diagnosis of lupus, I have also been removed from the National Marrow Donor Registry and can no longer donate blood products. It was while I was attending college at the University of Southern Maine that I signed up to be a part of the National Bone Marrow Donor Registry and became involved in donating platelet cells twice a week while I was in Portland.

Treatments are going well. My medication regimen now consists of eleven pills per day, which is much better than the original thirty two pills per day. They are on a schedule of one round in the morning and one round in the evening instead of having to remember five or six times per day. I only take my blood pressure twice a day now, sitting, instead of three times per day and three different readings each time: lying down, sitting up and standing as when I was first diagnosed. My blood work I have stretched out to having about once a month and the values remain within normal range for the most part. I am back standing and walking on my own and no longer dependent on a wheelchair or walker. I take great pride in being able to climb stairs on my own. I no longer have to sit a chair in the bathtub to take a shower, am able to drive by myself, go shopping and walk along the beach and area boardwalks in the evenings.

I am continuing to gain strength but a lot is dependent on the day. I still get tired easily and can only push myself so far before I have to crash for a nap. I determined that I am no different than anyone else in that respect because we all have our limits and everyone is different. If I do have 'big plans' I generally try to save my energy up either the day before or that morning if the plans are in the afternoon. Believe me, that becomes easier with time. When I first found out that I could do things again I was trying to cram everything I could into a day. I did not realize, at the time, that it would take about two days of doing nothing to recuperate from such activity! I wanted to do it all and I wanted to do it immediately. One of my greatest accomplishments was gaining the independence and ability to drive again.

A lot of my time during the day is spent writing, reading, cooking, arts and crafts projects and working on regaining strength, endurance as well as more independence. I am able to go out in the sun after 4pm so I frequent the beach for sunset.

My summers are now filled with some adventure. I am able to travel to Maine, for up to three months, to escape the heat and humidity of Tampa Bay, Florida. I am established to the point that I continue to receive blood work, have had intravenous treatments, and my doctor in Maine is in contact with my hematologist in Florida. This allows me the opportunity to visit with family and friends, be more active because the effects of the weather are not so dramatic for me and relax by the lake.

In stark contrast to my thirtieth birthday's chemotherapy cocktail running through my veins, about twenty minutes of my thirty-first birthday was spent parasailing, 1200 feet, above the Gulf of Mexico. It was amazing, just drifting along in the sky and admiring the beauty of my surroundings.

Children are not (biologically) in my future. I do not spend my time worrying about getting married, who it will be or even if it will happen. Life is too short to spend my time worrying and I have learned that God works not only in His own time but for the greater good. I have no right to place demands on what I believe I *need* when I am just beginning to figure out what direction I am being led. Children will always be a part of my life, through my work, and I am actually at peace with that thought. I know that if I allow the experience to play itself out I can only hope to make a difference in their lives but, with undeniable certainty, they will make a difference in mine.

I do not believe that my *life's purpose* is leading me back to the direction of nursing or medical school. Although I loved the work that I did and I learned a great deal from it, there is so much more that I have to share and in order to fully develop the gifts that

I have been given; a different venue and variety of options must be pursued.

I now have a *Bucket List*. Not because I plan on checking out of here anytime soon; however, this journey has most certainly changed my priorities in life. I would love to see the Smoky Mountains; continue to travel around the country and start hiking and camping (in a tent) again. I am also in the process of looking into what it would take to audit some college level classes and start a foundation of my own. Whatever life brings my way, I now realize that I have the strength to improvise, adapt and overcome not only the day to day challenges but doing so while focusing on the greater picture.

Never did I believe that I was one that would be remotely interested in public speaking but I believe that I have a story to share that others can learn from. My journey has been the tool used to teach me undeniable *life lessons* and by spreading my wings to envelop the experience I can be the instrument used to teach others. What has taken me years to learn may not be so for someone else if I am able to share this journey. It has taken me quite a while to comprehend that my journey will and already to some extent has worked out for a greater good, that this has actually been a gift that I am blessed to receive. With my words, my voice and my actions I will always be moving forward and praying that I can help others to do the same.

For I know the thoughts
I think toward you, says the LORD,
thoughts of peace and not of evil,
to give you a future and a hope.

Jeremiah 29:11

~ *Scripture Reference* ~

The following scriptures were all referenced in *The Dream* as well as *Getting by* and are provided here for your greater insight into my thoughts and feelings at the time. Each of the following versus are from the New King James Version of translation:

For by grace you have been saved through faith, and that not of yourselves; it is the gift of God, not of works, lest anyone should boast. For we are His workmanship, created in Christ Jesus for good works, which God prepared beforehand that we should walk in them.

Ephesians 2: 8 - 10

"For God so loved the world that He have His only begotten Son, that whoever believes in Him should not perish but have everlasting life."

John 3: 16

My brethren, count it all joy when you fall into various trials, knowing that the testing of your faith produces patience. But let patience have its perfect work, that you may be perfect and complete, lacking nothing.

James 1: 2 - 4

"Let not your heart be troubled; you believe in God, believe also in Me. In my Father's house are many mansions; if it were not so, I would have told you. I go to prepare a place for you. And if I go and prepare a place for you, I will come again and receive you to Myself; that where I am, there you may be also. And where I go you know, and the way you know. Thomas said to Him, "Lord, we do not know where You are going, and how can we know the way?" Jesus said to him, *"I am the way, the truth, and the life. No one comes to the Father except through Me."*

John 14: 1 - 6

Be anxious for nothing, but in everything by prayer and supplication, with thanksgiving, let your requests be made known to God; and the peace of God, which surpasses all understanding, will guard your hearts and minds through Christ Jesus.

Philippians 4: 6, 7

Seeing that we have a great High Priest who has passed through the heavens, Jesus the Son of God, let us hold fast our confession. For we do not have a High Priest who cannot sympathize with our weaknesses, but was in all points tempted as we are, yet without sin.

Hebrews 4: 14, 15

The LORD the Shepherd of His People
A Psalm of David

The LORD is my shepherd;
I shall not want.
He makes me to lie down in green pastures;
He leads me beside the still waters.
He restores my soul;
He leads me in the paths of righteousness
For His name's sake.
Yea, thought I walk through the valley of the shadow of death,
I will fear no evil;
For You are with me;
Your rod and Your staff, they comfort me.
You prepare a table for me in the presence of my enemies;
You anoint my head with oil;
My cup runs over.
Surely goodness and mercy shall follow me
All the days of my life;
And I will dwell in the house of the LORD
Forever.

23rd Psalm

And we know that all things work together for good to those who love God, to those who are the called according to His purpose.

Romans 8: 28

~ *Definition of Terms* ~

Acute Renal Failure - Temporary loss of kidney function

ANA - Antinuclear Antibody found in individuals whose immune system is prone to cause inflammation against its own cells

Autoimmune disease - An illness that occurs when the immune system attacks its own body's cells

Avascular Necrosis - A condition caused by poor blood supply to the bone, eventually leading to bone death

Barbiturates - Central nervous system depressants used as sedatives or hypnotics.

C-diff - Clostridium Difficile Colitis is the most common cause of infection of the colon.

Colitis - Inflammation of the inner lining of the colon.

Congestive Heart Failure - A condition in which the pumping of the heart is inadequate to meet the needs of the body.

Cushing's Syndrome - A hormone disorder caused by prolonged exposure to high levels of cortisol.

Debridement - The act of removing dead, adherent or contaminated tissue from an area

Hematologist - A physician who is specifically trained in the diagnosis, treatment and prevention of diseases dealing with the blood and bone marrow.

Hematuria - Blood in the urine.

Hypertension - Elevated blood pressure, usually a reading exceeding 140 over 90 mmHg.

IVC Filter - A filter placed in the inferior vena cava to prevent blood clots from going to the lungs.

Lupus - a chronic inflammatory disease that can affect various parts of the body, especially the skin, joints, blood and kidneys.

MRI - Magnetic Resonance Imaging. A specially designed radiology technique that uses magnetism, radio waves and a computer to produce images of internal structures of the body.

Nephrologist - A physician who is specifically trained in the diagnosis, treatment and prevention of diseases dealing with the kidneys.

Pancreatitis - Inflammation of the pancreas.

Rheumatologist - A specialist in the treatment of disorders having to do with connective tissue.

SLE - Systemic Lupus Erythematosus. A chronic inflammatory condition caused by the autoimmune disease lupus and is not contained to a specific area such as the skin.

TEE - Transesophageal Echocardiogphy uses ultrasound waves to produce images of the heart chambers, valves and surrounding structures.

Third Spacing - Accumulation of fluids in the space between the skin and connective tissue.

~ *Notes by the Reader* ~

86   MOVING FORWARD

Made in the USA
Charleston, SC
07 January 2010